The Hormone Reset Diet

The Ultimate Guide to Heal Your Metabolism, Balance Your Hormones, and Lose Up to 5 Pounds In 7 Days

© Copyright 2014 by Lucy Branson - All rights reserved.

This document is geared towards providing exact and reliable information in regards to the topic and issue covered. The publication is sold with the idea that the publisher is not required to render accounting, officially permitted, or otherwise, qualified services. If advice is necessary, legal or professional, a practiced individual in the profession should be ordered.

- From a Declaration of Principles which was accepted and approved equally by a Committee of the American Bar Association and a Committee of Publishers and Associations.

In no way is it legal to reproduce, duplicate, or transmit any part of this document in either electronic means or in printed format. Recording of this publication is strictly prohibited and any storage of this document is not allowed unless with written permission from the publisher. All rights reserved.

The information provided herein is stated to be truthful and consistent, in that any liability, in terms of inattention or otherwise, by any usage or abuse of any policies, processes, or directions contained within is the solitary and utter responsibility of the recipient reader. Under no circumstances will any legal responsibility or blame be held against the publisher for any reparation, damages, or monetary loss due to the information herein, either directly or indirectly.

Respective authors own all copyrights not held by the publisher.

The information herein is offered for informational purposes solely, and is universal as so. The presentation of the information is without contract or any type of guarantee assurance.

The trademarks that are used are without any consent, and the publication of the trademark is without permission or backing by the trademark owner. All trademarks and brands within this book are for clarifying purposes only and are the owned by the owners themselves, not affiliated with this document.

Table of Contents

Introduction — 4
Chapter 1: Your Hormones — 6
Chapter 2: Why Should You Do A Hormone Reset Diet? — 12
Chapter 3: The Hormone Reset Diet — 14
Chapter 4: The Hormone Reset Recipes — 22
Chapter 5: Faq — 28
Conclusion — 31

Introduction

I want to thank you and congratulate you for downloading the book, *"The Hormone Reset Diet: The Ultimate Guide to Heal Your Metabolism, Balance Your Hormones, and Lose Up to 5 Pounds In 7 Days"*.

You and I, as well as the dozens of other women who also made the conscious decision to take action against their weight gain through this book, have something in common — you've experienced how difficult it is to lose weight after several (and I do mean several) diet and exercise attempts.

Weight loss has probably been the oldest struggle in the book for the majority of the female population. Book after book has been released, claiming to be the true cure for fat and obesity, but only a few really deliver what they promised. Is it because the book programs weren't effective? Is it because the dieting and exercising programs found in these books weren't done properly? Or is it because numerous authors have overlooked one, single factor that may have appeared trivial but, in truth, has been the culprit for women's mood swings, changing bodily functions, abnormal eating habits and slowed metabolism?

Personally, I'm betting my money on the last question and you should too. Hormones have never really been the core topic for a weight loss book because, even though, medically, they have been known to affect weight under certain circumstances, they weren't viewed as a major player, unlike eating right (dieting) and training your body (exercising).

This is exactly what we're going to explore in this book! Hormones may not have been key topics in several weight loss books but, now, we're going to get to the bottom of how you can beat flab by resetting your hormones. We're also going to learn more about the different processes and recipes involved in Hormone Reset and it doesn't stop there.

Thanks again for downloading this book, I hope you enjoy it!

Chapter 1: Your Hormones

Before we go to the good stuff, let's first understand the facts.

When a woman's hormones are out of sync, it can lead to several effects on our body, which includes the build-up of fat. If you have extra handles on you, chances are, you have one or two of the following hormonal imbalances:

• High Estrogen

• Low Testosterone

• High Insulin

• High Cortisol

• High Leptin

• Deficient Growth Hormone

• Deficient Thyroid Hormone

Estrogen

Estrogen and fat have a very complicated relationship. Fat isn't just a big blob of lard sitting on your hips. It's a vital part of your hormone system since one of its major jobs is to produce estrogen. An enzyme called aromatase contained in fat tissues converts testosterone to estrogen. There are loads more where estrogen came from. This is just one source of it that's important to know in weight loss/weight gain situations.

It can also work the other way around. Estrogen overload can exaggerate hypothyroid issues, slowing down your metabolism and causing you to gain weight. Another possibility is that high levels of estrogen promote fat gain through the prevention of using these fats as energy.

Like what I said, it's a complicated relationship but more certain than not, estrogen is a key hormone to weight gain or weight loss.

Testosterone

Testosterone is a hormone found in both men and women. It's the hormone responsible for increased muscle mass, bone density and metabolism. A low level of testosterone can lead to an increased risk for depression, low sex drive, obesity and osteoporosis

Insulin

Here's how the normal process goes: after we eat our bodies release insulin which tells our muscles, livers and fat cells to take up the sugar and fat and remove it from our bloodstream since it could be toxic for the body. However, the liver and muscle cells have a limited capacity to store glucose (or sugar) hence they shut their "doors" when excessive carbs are consumed on a daily basis even with the pancreas releasing enough amounts of insulin. Having nowhere else to go, the sugar in our blood gets sent to fat cells. The result? I think you know...

With the "doors" shut, the pancreas will release more insulin to normalize blood sugar levels. With more insulin released glucose levels can be brought down to a safe level again...at least for a while. Over time, fasting blood sugar levels start to creep up and the entire process will result to insulin resistance.

Cortisol

When we're stressed, several hormones are released. This includes adrenalin, which gives us instant energy, corticotrophin releasing hormone or CRH and cortisol. Adrenalin and CRH, at high levels, cause a decrease in appetite. This effect, however, doesn't usually last very long. Cortisol, on the other hand, works in a very different way. Its main function is to help our body replenish after the stress has gone. It "hangs around" a bit longer and elevated levels of this cause an increase in our appetite, driving us to eat more.

Leptin

Leptin is another hormone secreted by fat cells. Its main role is to send signals to the brain, telling it that our bodies have enough energy stored up and that we don't need to eat. If you have increased amounts of this, your brain should be telling your body that it's had enough, right? Yes, that is what's supposed to happen. In the case of obesity, an increased leptin has been found in the bloodstream but the problem is the brain doesn't recognize it. This state is called leptin resistance.

But, why in the world is our brain blinded when insane amounts of leptin are already in our body? It's because of another hormone called insulin. It could be one of the reasons why our brain is not picking up on the signal leptin is giving off. Darn you insulin!

Growth Hormone

Isn't growth hormone supposed to make you grow? So, low levels of it will make you small?

Yes, generally, that's the idea. Children with a growth hormone deficiency are, generally, smaller than their peers but it isn't only the growth that it's responsible for. One of its functions is to regulate our bodies' metabolism. Adults with a deficiency have been found to have high levels of fat as well as cholesterol in their bodies. Many would link this to unhealthy eating but even if an adult eat well but has ADGH (Adult Growth Hormone Deficiency), similar findings will be observed.

Thyroid Hormone

Thyroid hormones also play a major role in our body in connection with weight loss or weight gain. One of its functions is to, basically, regulate our calorie intake. A deficiency in this hormone results in a low basal metabolic rate and a difficulty to lose extra weight. Sounds familiar to you?

There are more...

It doesn't stop there too. This is just an overview of the many hormones involved in the process of weight gain. Am I saying that there are more hormones and not just the seven already mentioned? YES.

The whole thing sounds so alarming, doesn't it? "What other hormones are out of whack in my body?" you might be asking but don't go running to your doctor to get some tests done just yet.

Hormonal imbalances, though very scientific sounding, are not medical issues but, more often, they are a nutritional issue.

It is true and it is surprising. The very thing that you're snacking on right now may be causing your body, as well as your hormones, to go crazy on food. So, put the snack down slowly and let's continue.

I'm saying this not because I want to scare you to do a Hormone Reset (well, maybe I am just a little) but I'm saying this so your eyes can be opened to the facts. It isn't only diet and exercises that will help us lose a couple of pounds. They're good on their own but the idea that I want to leave you is this:

A more effective approach to weight loss is by controlling or managing the very things that affect the inside of our body these are hormones.

Chapter 2: Why should you do a hormone reset diet?

OK so you're probably skeptical and you're asking me this question. You're asking me for reasons why you, or anyone else for that matter, need to reset their hormones.

Fair enough and I have just the answers for your question:

You need a change.

If you're tired of doing diet after diet, and exercise after exercise without getting the results you're expecting, then what have you got to lose? You need a change and this could be it.

Your body needs it.

I can't stress this enough. The main reason why many diets and exercises fail is because they've neglected one big factor and that's hormones. Learning how to control your hormones will give you a new perspective on how your body works. And, knowing how your body works will give you fresher ideas on how you can keep it healthy.

You'll feel loads better about yourself.

I know that exercise also promises the same thing with the release of endorphins (the happy hormone) but that's just one.

Imagine how fabulous you're going to feel if you've reset all the six hormones we're focusing on.

You'll lose weight

This is our main goal, right? Aside from being healthy and being educated on how your body works, you'll also lose weight, which is what we're all trying to do!

Because you are targeting what's happening on the inside of your body, you're not going against any natural reaction with will power. All you really need is to cook the suggested recipes and eat!

Chapter 3: The hormone reset diet

The fundamental principle of resetting your hormones is to ensure that your mind and body will be coordinated properly to allow healthy cell metabolism which will then result in weight loss and better health. The hormone reset diet dictates that in a period of 3 days, there will be specific changes to your dietary program. In order to reset your estrogen hormones, gut bacteria and liver, you need to eliminate alcohol and meat in your diet. Every 3 days specific foods that wreck your metabolism need to be changed into healthier alternatives to reset the imbalanced hormones in the body. Once the hormones are reset, your mind and body will begin to function in harmony and you'll start to truly feel good about yourself.

Only 3 days?

Well the minimum time allowed for a metabolic hormone reset is three days. However, in some cases, a 5-days reset is allowed especially for people who shouldn't have immediate dietary changes. Still, 3 days is the ideal amount of time because it completes the cycle of resetting the 7 metabolic hormones in 21 days.

How is Hormone Reset diet done?

The goal of the hormone reset diet is to synchronize the 7 hormones of metabolism: estrogen, insulin, leptin, Cortisol, thyroid hormones, serotonin, and testosterone. Here is an overview of the hormone reset (every 3 days).

- No meat and alcohol: you are a meat eater or not, this reset is important to everyone. Eliminating alcohol and red meat in your diet resets your estrogen levels in the body.

- No sugar: After 3 days of not eating red meat and no alcohol, eliminate or in some cases, reduce sugar in your food intake to reset your insulin hormone and eradicate sugar cravings.

- Less Fruits: After another 3 days reset leptin hormone by not eating fruits for 3 days.

- No Caffeine: Caffeine increases Cortisol in the bloodstream so eliminating caffeine resets Cortisol levels and reduces your susceptibility to stress.

- No Grains: Not eating grains for 3 days resets your thyroid hormones which are essential in controlling and resetting leptin and insulin levels.

- No dairy products: Resets growth hormones and improves insulin

- No toxins: Detoxifying resets testosterone levels which aids in proper reset of insulin, thyroid hormones, estrogen and leptin.

After 21 days, you will notice that your metabolism transformed you from within and you will feel better than you have ever felt before. You will no longer have to constantly battle weight gain and stress and you will have better sleep. You'll also have better sex with your partner.

The claim behind the hormone diet is that most of the weight problems result from hormonal imbalance. Dr. Natasha Turner, the author of this said program, explains how the rise and fall of specific levels of hormone in the blood can cause accumulation and storage of excessive body fat. Not only does it cause weight gain, it also contributes to a lagging libido, health problems, sluggishness, sugar cravings and stress.

Dr. Turner encourages a 2-weeks detox and a lifestyle change to solve hormonal imbalance with a strict observation of

Mediterranean-style diet with additional supplements. She believes that with this hormone diet plan, you can transform your health and energy levels and eliminate excess pounds in as early as one week.

The Food Plan:

The other term for the hormone diet is Glyci-Med which is a combination of foods with low GI (Glycemic Index) and the traditional Mediterranean diet. These foods do not cause rapid boost in sugar levels and so they don't increase the cravings.

Here is a list of the foods that are recommended under the Glyci-Med diet:

- Vegetables
- Fruits that are low in sugar
- Flax seeds
- Chia seeds
- Lean protein like eggs and chicken breasts
- Fish
- Olive oil
- Nuts
- Quinoa
- Unsaturated fats and oil like canola
- Whole grains like brown rice and buckwheat

Foods that are not recommended under the Glyci-Med diet:

- Alcohol
- Processed meat
- Caffeine
- Saturated fat
- Fried foods
- Foods high in GI like pasta and white bread
- Artificial sweeteners
- Peanuts
- Full fat dairy products

Meal frequency

80 percent of the time, food choices are healthy and can be taken in every 3-4 hours. There is one or two "cheat meals" a week

It is never easy to drastically change your eating patterns and habits. The hormone diet restricts a lot of food products that a person can easily get attached to. You will be required to quit sugar, alcohol, caffeine, most oils, gluten and dairy for 2- 3 weeks. This may cause problems to some people especially those who have a habit of taking these foods at frequent intervals on a daily basis. The bodys pH balance also needs to be monitored. A series of tests also needs to be done to ensure safety and well-being of the practitioners especially on the first stage of the hormone diet. These tests include saliva, urine and blood tests to check hormone levels. Finally, the diet plan also recommends supplements like calcium, vitamin D3, magnesium, Omega 3 and multivitamins.

Drawbacks:

The hormone diet is a big adjustment for people who were used to eating prepared snacks and meals because the foods need to be prepared at home. Giving up alcohol and soda for example is also very difficult to do because not everyone likes to drink green tea.

Shopping and cooking: Organic foods are recommended. There will be a one week sample recipes provided and these are relatively simple. Options are also limited if you are not comfortable about the idea of foods on the diet plan and how they are supposed to be prepared.

What sort of exercise is needed?

Exercise activities like yoga, cardio, strength training, and interval training are advised for 30 minutes every day.

Are dietary preferences and restrictions allowed?

For those who are into gluten-free diet, the restriction is only up for 2 weeks. After 2 weeks, gluten is allowed in minimal amounts. Dr. Turner advises that it is good to avoid white rice and white bread and just eat their brown variants because they are healthier. And for those who are eating vegetables and lean protein, like the vegetarians and vegans, they have nothing to worry about because the diet is composed mainly of vegetables and some protein which works well for them. Any foods that may have a negative effect on the body after the detox phase need to be avoided.

Is it cheap?

Organic foods are more expensive than the foods that we normally buy in the supermarket. You also need to buy hormone tests which may not be covered by your insurance and some recommended supplements. So if you cannot afford additional expenses, hormone diet as recommended by Dr. Turner may not be a good option for you. The good news is, even without the tests, you can still finish the hormone reset diet plan in 2-3 weeks. The result will more likely be the same without the hormone tests because you can definitely feel the difference after the detox period.

Is it effective in weight loss?

Yes, it is effective in weight loss. The dietary plan consists of foods that are low in calories. Other positive effects of the Glyci-Med diet according to practitioner testimonies are:

- Better sleep patterns
- Healthy and glowing skin
- Healthier and vibrant hair
- Reduced stress
- Better sex with their partner
- and weight loss

However, some scientists believe that supplements are not really advisable if you are on organic diet. Organic diet is really healthy but there are still natural alternatives to good health and weight loss that are cheaper.

Glyci-Med diet or a low-carb diet in general offers rewarding results and benefits to most people. It helps improve health conditions like heart disease, hypertension and diabetes.

Chapter 4: The hormone reset recipes

This eBook about hormone reset diet will not be complete without sample recipes. Beginners need to know how the food is prepared and which ingredients are best used for one particular meal. The recipes provided here are very easy to make and the ingredients can be found easily in the supermarkets.

Blueberry smoothie with goat yogurt

Ingredients:

- Frozen blueberries (1/2 cup)
- Frozen banana (1/2 cup)
- Plain goat yogurt (1/2 cup)
- Chia seeds (1 tbsp)
- Whey protein isolate (1 serving)
- Water (1/2 cup)

Directions:

Using a blender, mix the purée and all the ingredients together until the consistency is smooth.

Lettuce wraps and Crispy Chicken

Ingredients:

- 4-5 ounces Chicken breast (boneless and skinless)
- Small Lettuce head
- Cucumber (1/4 cup — diced)
- Red bell pepper (1/4 cup- diced)
- Unpeeled green apple (diced)
- Low-fat Greek yogurt (1/4 cup)
- Red onion (1 tbsp — finely chopped)
- Virgin olive oil (2 tsp)
- Pepper
- Salt

Directions:

- Put the lettuce away and mix all the ingredients together in a medium-sized bowl.
- Put the bowl in the chiller and leave it there for at least an hour.
- After one hour, scoop the chicken mixture and carefully place inside each lettuce leaf.
- Roll each leaf into cylinders.
- Serve.

Tropical Smoothie

Ingredients:

- Water (2 cups)
- Peeled Mango (cubed)
- Banana (peeled)
- Raw Baby Spinach (2-3 cups)

Directions:

- Using a blender, combine all the ingredients together until consistency is smooth.

Pecan Candy

Ingredients:

- Pecans (2 cups)
- Yacon syrup (2 tbsp)
- Salt (1/2 tsp)
- Olive oil (1 tbsp)

Directions:

- Using a large bowl, mix all the ingredients together.
- Set the oven at 350oF.
- Put the mixture in a baking dish (9x13)
- Bake the mixture for 15 minutes.

- Let it cool for 5 min outside the oven.
- Serve and enjoy.

Mac and Cheese Prosciutto with Caramelized Onion

Ingredients:

- 1/2 cup Parmesan cheese (grated)
- 1/4 tsp. of black pepper
- 1/4 cup of goat cheese
- 1 clean and trimmed head of cauliflower head
- 1 cup of heavy cream
- 1 medium diced onion
- 1 cup of sharp shredded cheddar cheese
- 2 tbsp. of olive oil
- 3 cloves of garlic (large, minced)
- 4 tbsp. of butter
- 6 oz. of diced Prosciutto (cooked until crisp)

Steps:

- Preheat the oven to 350 degrees.
- Add water about an inch high in a big pot with cover.
- Add the cauliflower in the pot and steam until tender.

- Once the cauliflower is tender, remove the pot from the heat.
- Drain the water and do not remove the cauliflower in the pot yet to release the excess water.
- Transfer cauliflower in a dish and gently break the cauliflower apart, using a fork
- Place a pan over medium heat.
- Heat the olive oil and half of the butter in the pan.
- Add the onions.
- Sauté until the mixture takes the color of caramel.
- Remove the onion and set aside.
- Add the garlic and the remaining half of butter in the pan that you used for the onions.
- Sauté until you can smell the garlic and the butter melts.
- Add the parmesan cheese and heavy cream.
- Stir until the parmesan melts and let the sauce boil.
- Add the black pepper, cheddar cheese, and goat cheese.
- Mix until the cheese melts and blends in the sauce nicely.

- Lower the heat. Simmer for 5 minutes and let the sauce thicken.
- Pour the cheese and let it evenly cover the cauliflower.
- Add the caramelized onions on top of the cheese sauce.
- Add the prosciutto on top of the onion.
- Sprinkle the rest of the cheese that you did not melt.
- Place in the oven and let it bake for 15 minutes.
- Serve and enjoy!

Chapter 5: FAQ

Do I need to exercise while on this program?

Not necessarily but you'll get better results when you do exercise. It doesn't have to be an hour of cross fit every day. Like

I said earlier, you just have to make sure that your body is moving — stretches will do, basic yoga poses will do, walking to the nearest park will do and jogging for 30mins will, definitely do.

Find an exercise that fits your time. There's no specific exercise requirement, remember that.

How will I be feeling while on the hormone reset?

The hormone reset will be managing your hormones so it's highly likely that your mood swings and your cravings will be under control. How you feel will be entirely up to how your body is reacting. It's different from one individual to another.

How much weight will I lose?

I've mentioned this earlier. This will again, depend on how your body reacts to the program. You can lose as much as 15lbs in just 3 weeks but, another scenar10 is that, you may not lose much at all.

DONT PANIC! My advice is to keep at it so you can, thoroughly, reset your hormones and then you can measure your metrics right after to really tell if it was effective or not. You might just be surprised about what you'll discover with your results!

What should I do if I have cravings?

Remember when I said that you need to exercise your will power at least for the first few days? It's no-negotiable. If you're experiencing cravings, simply don't give in to them. Instead, replace them with something that you CAN eat during your hormone reset. Snack on something healthy that doesn't go beyond what's inhibited.

Will I gain weight after I do the program?

It's not impossible, let me tell you that. The thought of reentry after 21 days of diet restrictions is very heavenly. Do go overboard as you may cause one or two hormonal imbalances. Then, you're back to ground zero if this happens and this means that you're probably going to gain back the weight you lost.

Is the program safe to do?

Yes it is. If you're feeling extra anxious about it, go and check with your doctor or with your nutritionist. Nonetheless, please remember that this program is just like any diet out there (like the paleo diet or gluten free diet as you may notice with the recipes). The main difference is it's merely geared towards resetting hormones and it's not just about eating well and losing weight.

Conclusion

Hi there. I hope that you found this book helpful. I just wanted to add this section in so I can sneak in a few words about resetting hormones.

The struggle with weight is real! No matter what diet or exercise we do, we always find it difficult to lose a certain amount of weight given the little amount of time (and sometimes resources) that we have every day. Am I preaching to the congregation yet? If I hit a note, that's because I've gone through it myself. I know how difficult it is to lose weight if you don't even have time to exercise or if you don't have enough resources to prepare and eat the right kind of food.

This is why I made the program customizable. I want you to add in what you can contribute. You don't have to, strictly, follow the recipes I stated here. Make it your own. As for exercising, you can do without it for this program but I encourage you to have 30mins of moving every day. It could be basic stretches, walking, jogging or what have you. Just make sure that you move your body 30mins a day.

Also, don't be intimidated by success stories you read online saying that the program worked for them and they lost 1 million pounds in just 3 weeks (an exaggeration, of course). Though we are correcting the same kind of hormones, our body can react differently to the program causing you to lose weight slowly or drastically. Trust the process and trust how your body feels. Go through with it and see if you can note any difference. If you can, that means that something is happening and you just need to keep at it for 21 days.

What I'm saying may sound easy to say but hard to do. That's because it is. This is the hard truth to it. Even if you're moving 30mins a day and you've found a way to customize the meals to fit your resources, it's still going to take a much of your time and effort but the good news is, there's a pot of gold at the end of the rainbow and I'm really hoping that you find your pit of gold soon!

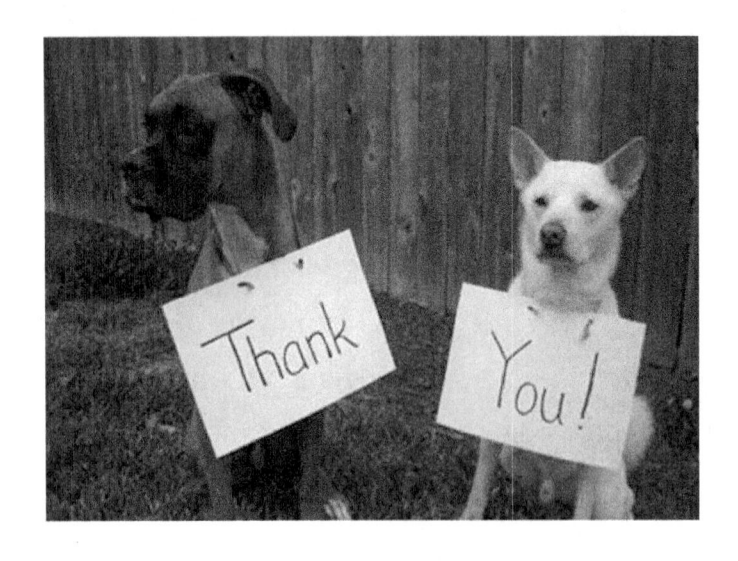

Finally, if you enjoyed this book, then I'd like to ask you for a favor, would you be kind enough to leave a review for this book on Amazon? It'd be greatly appreciated!

Please, leave a review for this book on Amazon!

Thank you and good luck!

Printed in Great Britain
by Amazon